HOW TO GET RID OF HEAVY WEIGHT

THE BEST WAY TO REDUCE CHOLESTEROL

JERRY E. CLEMENT

2

Disclaimer Note

This book is only intended to provide knowledge that is relevant to daily me.Every effort has been made to provide accurate, current, trustworthy, and comprehensive information. In no way should you take this as medical advice; instead, you should speak with your physician.

TABLE OF CONTENT

INTRODUCTION

This archive concerns weight reduction, an issue interminably on many individuals' psyches. Most everybody needs to be thin and conditioned, however actually it is far more straightforward to put on weight than to lose it. In the accompanying pages reasons for weight gain are surveyed, alongside various justifications for why individuals ought to give the work important to decrease their weight to suggested levels. Having given inspiration to a get-healthy plan, we close with a review of weight reduction strategies, and ideas for accomplishing long-lasting solid weight reduction. Begin currently by turning the page.

CHAPTER 1

DIET AND NUTRITION

What is a solid eating regimen? What does a solid eating regimen resemble?"

A solid eating regimen favors regular, natural food sources over pre-bundled feasts and tidbits. It is adjusted, implying that it furnishes your body with every one of the supplements and minerals it necessities to work best. It stresses plant-based food sources — particularly products of the soil — over creature food varieties. It contains a lot of protein. It is low in sugar and salt. It consolidates "solid fats" including fish, olive oil and other plant-inferred oils.

Here are a couple of instances of quality dinners for weight reduction. For breakfast, a bowl of wheat drops with cut strawberries and pecans with nonfat milk. For lunch, a turkey sandwich on wheat with vegetables and an olive oil and vinegar dressing. For supper, a salmon steak on a bed of spinach.

You don't need to remove snacks to eat a sound eating routine, all things considered. Sound snacks for weight reduction incorporate almonds or pistachios, string cheddar with an apple, Greek yogurt or a banana with peanut butter.

Recollect that the best eating regimen is the one you'll adhere to, so don't rush out and purchase a lot of "wellbeing food varieties" that you realize you won't ever eat.

What's the best eating regimen?
There is no single eating regimen that nutritionists have considered "the best."
In any case, there are a few

styles of eating that specialists either have intended for ideal wellbeing or have seen to be sound when consumed customarily by various individuals all over the planet. Such styles of eating will generally share a couple of things practically speaking — they will quite often be plant-based consumes less calories, they stress sound fats, no basic sugars and low sodium, and they favor regular food sources over the profoundly handled passage common of a large part of the Western eating regimen.

For instance, the Mediterranean style diet gets its name from the food varieties accessible to different societies situated around the Mediterranean

Ocean. It intensely accentuates insignificantly handled natural products, vegetables, vegetables, nuts and entire grains. It contains moderate measures of yogurt, cheddar, poultry and fish. Olive oil is its essential cooking fat. Red meat and food sources with added sugars are just eaten sparingly. Other than being a successful weight reduction technique, eating a Mediterranean style diet is connected to a lower chance of coronary illness, diabetes, discouragement and a few types of cancer.Experts fostered the

Run diet (Dietary Ways to deal with Hypertension)

 explicitly as a heart-solid routine. The blend of food types contained in the eating regimen appear to cooperate particularly successfully to bring down circulatory strain and reduce the hazard of cardiovascular breakdown. The critical highlights of Run are low cholesterol and soaked fats, bunches of magnesium, calcium, fiber and potassium, and practically no red meat and sugar. Obviously, that is similar to a rundown of food varieties like those of the

Mediterranean eating routine — entire grains, vegetables, organic products, fish, poultry, nuts and olive oil.

As its name infers, the

 MIND diet (Mediterranean-Run diet Mediation for Neurodegenerative Deferral) was planned by specialists to take components from the Mediterranean and Run counts calories that appeared to give advantages to cerebrum wellbeing and fight off dementia and mental degradation. By and by, it is basically the same as both the Mediterranean and Run slims down, however it puts more grounded accentuation on verdant green vegetables and berries, and less accentuation on leafy foods.

As of late, the Nordic eating regimen has arisen as both a weight reduction and wellbeing support diet. In view of Scandinavian eating designs, the Nordic eating routine is weighty on fish, apples, pears, entire grains like rye and oats, and cold-environment vegetables including cabbage, carrots and cauliflower. Studies have upheld its utilization both in forestalling stroke and in weight reduction.

They're all great for your heart, they all consist of regular natural food varieties and they all contain a lot of plant-based dishes. Eating for your wellbeing — particularly your heart wellbeing — by taking on components from these eating regimens is a savvy method for shedding pounds.

How could feast plans influence your weight?

A few specialists suggest eating feasts prior in the day to control weight, and some proof backs that up. For instance, a recent report found that eating later in the day expanded craving and fat stockpiling, and diminished hunger, decreasing chemical levels and fat consumption. To eat feasts prior in the day, one methodology is eating either two huge dinners each day (an enormous breakfast and a second huge dinner in midafternoon) or if nothing else having a third feast that closes by 5 p.m.

CHAPTER 2

BODY WEIGHT LOSS EXERCISE

Eating a sound eating regimen doesn't guarantee

that you will get more fit. Your weight is a harmony between the calories you take in and the calories you consume. You will get thinner on the off chance that you consume off additional calories than you take in, and you will put on weight assuming you eat a bigger number of calories than you consume off. You can shed pounds by eating less, however adding active work permits you to consume a larger number of calories than slimming down alone.

Any weight reduction plan that incorporates ordinary activity isn't just more fruitful — it's likewise better. By eating a sound eating routine and working out, you're keeping your bones, muscles, and heart solid. You additionally bring down your possibilities of getting specific medical issues, similar to hypertension and diabetes.

As opposed to abstaining from excessive food intake, center around sound propensities, such as eating more products of the soil and working out. Regardless of whether you get more fit, you will be better and you will feel and look good as well.

Beside counting calories, practicing is one of the most widely recognized procedures utilized by those attempting to shed additional pounds.

As well as assisting you with getting in shape, practice has numerous different advantages, including further developed state of mind, more grounded bones, and a decreased gamble of numerous ongoing illnesses

Here are the best activities for weight reduction.

1.Walking

Squeezing strolling into your everyday routine is simple. To add more moves toward your day, have a go at strolling during your mid-day break, using the stairwell at work, or taking your canine for additional strolls.

To begin, it means to stroll for 30 minutes 3-4 times each week. You can steadily build the length or recurrence of your strolls as you become more fit.

.2 Jogging or running

Despite the fact that they appear to be comparable, the key contrast is that a running speed is by and large between 4-6 mph (6.4-9.7 km/h), while a running speed is quicker than 6 mph (9.7 km/)

Additionally, investigations have discovered that

running and running can help copy instinctive fat, normally known as midsection fat. This sort of fat folds over your inside organs and has connections to different constant infections like coronary illness and diabetes .

Both running and running are extraordinary activities that should be possible anyplace and are not difficult to integrate into your week by week schedule. To begin, it means to run for 20-30 minutes 3-4 times each week.

Assuming you find running or running outside severe with your joints, take a stab at running on gentler surfaces like grass. Likewise, numerous treadmills have inherent padding, which might be simpler on your joints.

3 Weight preparation
Weight lifting is a famous decision for individuals hoping to get in shape.

A 155-pound (70-kg) individual consumes approximately 108 calories each 30 minutes of powerlifting

Additionally, power lifting can assist you with developing fortitude and advanced muscle development, which can raise your resting metabolic rate (RMR), or the number of calories your body consumes.

Another investigation discovered that 24 weeks of powerlifting prompted a 9% expansion in metabolic rate among men, which compared to copying roughly 140 additional calories each day. Among ladies, the expansion in metabolic rate was almost 4%, or 50 additional calories each day ,

Furthermore, studies have shown that your body keeps on consuming calories numerous hours after a power lifting exercise, contrasted and high-impact workout

4Yoga
Yoga is a well known method for practicing and easing pressure.

While it's not usually considered a weight reduction workout, it consumes a decent measure of calories and offers numerous extra medical advantages that can advance weight reduction.

Harvard Wellbeing gauges that a 155-pound (70-kg) individual consumes around 144 calories each 30 minutes of rehearsing yoga

Moreover, the yoga bunch experienced enhancements in mental and actual prosperity.

Beside consuming calories, studies have demonstrated the way that yoga can show care and lessen feelings of anxiety.

Cycling
Cycling is in many cases promoted as a decent low-influence choice for oxygen consuming activity.

That is on the grounds that you can consume a

noteworthy number of calories while you're accelerating, particularly assuming you cycle past a relaxed speed.

CHAPTER 3

GETTING A GOOD REST AND SLEEP

Rest assumes an essential part in the sound working of our body and, in this way, absence of it can bring about a few medical problems like diabetes, hypertension, cardiovascular sickness, disabled mental capacity, and psychological wellness issues, among others. However, did you have at least some idea that rest likewise has an immediate

connection to weight reduction? "Various examinations have proposed that confined rest and unfortunate rest quality might prompt metabolic issues, weight gain, and an expanded gamble of heftiness and other persistent ailments,"
To help weight reduction, it is prescribed to rest for 7-9 hours, specialists say.

It makes a difference "forestall corpulence, and keep cortisol levels from turning out to be excessively high - one of the more clear reasons for weight gain and muscle loss".also,beneficial as it causes you to feel vigorous, consequently, going about as a persuasive device for enjoying an active work which is straightforwardly connected with weight reduction. Additionally, dozing early decreases the possibilities of late evening nibbling on low quality food/high fat and carbs snacks," dietitian Upasana Sharma.

CHAPTER 4

MAINTAIN YOUR WEIGHT LOSS

Being dynamic and picking good food sources can help you keep up with or accomplish a sound weight, feel more lively, and decline your possibilities of having other medical conditions. It's essential to pick food varieties wealthy in supplements and go for the gold 150 minutes of actual work each week.

The energy your body gets from the food sources and beverages you eat is estimated in calories. Your body needs a specific number of calories every day, contingent upon your action level and different elements, to keep up with your ongoing weight.

To shed pounds, practice more or eat less calories than is suggested. To put on weight, increment the quantity of calories you eat while keeping a moderate action level.

Attempt to follow a good dieting design wealthy in vegetables, organic products, entire grains, low-fat dairy, and lean proteins.

.

Eat good food

Eat more food sources with sound fats, like avocados and peanut butter.
In the event that you get full rapidly, eat regular, more modest dinners over the course of the day.
Add supplement thick bites like nuts, cheddar, and dried

natural products to your menu.

Eat with loved ones to make the experience more pleasant.

Remain dynamic to support your craving.

Exercise consistently

Practice and actual work are great for practically everybody including more seasoned grown-ups. Hold back nothing 150 minutes of moderate-power oxygen consuming action — buckling down to the point of raising your pulse and starting to perspire every week. You don't need to achieve this at the same time, rather, you can separate your movement throughout the span of seven days. On the off chance that you can't meet the objective immediately, attempt to be as actually dynamic as possible. Showing improvement over doing nothing by any means.

For grown-ups at each weight, maturing is related to muscle misfortune, which makes specific exercises troublesome. Being dynamic can assist more established grown-ups with keeping up with bulk and make it simpler to direct everyday exercises, partake in trips, drive, stay aware of grandkids, keep away from falls, and remain as autonomous as could be expected.

You don't have to burn through a huge load of cash joining a rec center or employing a fitness coach to get fit. Contemplate the sorts of proactive tasks that you appreciate, for instance, strolling, running, bicycling, planting, swimming, and moving. Indeed, even ordinary tasks, for example, vacuuming can give active work. While you're beginning with workout, attempt to remain inspired to routinely move your body. Then, at that point, increment the period of time you exercise or add another pleasant actually..